INTRODUCTION

Welcome to "Feminine Harmony: Nutrition and Well-being at Every Age," a guide designed to accompany you through the different phases of life with wisdom, well-being, and balance. This book is an ode to all women seeking to harmonize their diet with their body and spirit at every stage of life.

From the flourishing thirties to the blossoming wisdom of the sixties, each chapter of this book is an open window to tailored nutritional advice, science-based weight management strategies, and tips for optimal mental and physical well-being. We will address how the foods we choose not only influence our figure, but also our mood, our energy, and our longevity.

This book is not just a collection of recipes or diets; it's a life companion that guides you towards a better understanding of your body and its changing needs. With inspiring testimonials, accessible exercise programs, and balanced menus, prepare to embark on a journey towards a better version of yourself.

Understanding the Basics of Nutrition

Nutrition is the science that studies the interactions between food and living beings. For women, understanding these interactions is crucial for maintaining hormonal balance, managing weight, and aging healthily. This chapter breaks down macronutrients and micronutrients, and guides you through the art of reading food labels.

The Macronutrients: The Building Blocks of Our Diet
Proteins: Essential building blocks of our muscles, skin, enzymes, and hormones. Found in:
- Meat (chicken, beef, pork)
- Fish and seafood
- Legumes (lentils, chickpeas)
- Dairy products (cheese, yogurt)
- Eggs
- Nuts and seeds

Fats: Provide energy and are necessary for the production of our cells and hormones. Healthy sources include:
- Vegetable oils (olive, canola)
- Avocados
- Fatty fish (salmon, mackerel)
- Nuts and seeds
- Dark chocolate

Carbohydrates: Our main source of energy. It is important to choose complex carbohydrates for stable energy release:
- Whole grains (brown rice, quinoa, oats)
- Vegetables (broccoli, spinach, carrots)
- Fruits (apples, bananas, berries)
- Legumes

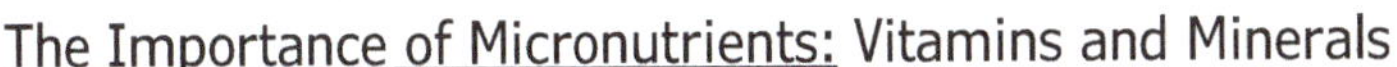

The Importance of Micronutrients: Vitamins and Minerals

Micronutrients are involved in almost all processes of our body. They are vital for our immune system, bone health, and overall well-being. For example:
Iron (important for oxygen transport and present in red meat, spinach, lentils)

Calcium (essential for bones and found in dairy products, tofu, almonds)

Vitamin D (crucial for bone health and immunity, present in fatty fish, egg yolks, or obtained through sun exposure)

Reading and Understanding Food Labels

Food labels are your window into the composition of your foods. Here's how to decipher them:

The Ingredients List: Ingredients are listed in decreasing order of quantity. Look for foods with natural and recognizable ingredients.

Nutritional Values: They indicate the amount of macronutrients, fiber, sugar, and salt. Opt for foods rich in protein and fiber, and low in added sugars and salt.

Nutritional Claims: Be wary of terms like "light," "sugar-free," or "high in fiber." They follow specific regulations but can be misleading.

Hormonal Balance and Nutrition

Hormonal balance is a key factor in overall health in women. Hormones influence not only reproduction and metabolism but also mood and energy. Adequate nutrition can help regulate these delicate hormones.

Phytoestrogens: Allies of Hormonal Balance

Phytoestrogens are plant compounds that can mimic or modulate the activity of estrogens in the body. They are particularly useful during menopause to mitigate symptoms related to hormonal fluctuations.

Dietary Sources: Soy, flaxseed, legumes.

Healthy Fats: For Hormones and Beyond

Essential fatty acids, including omega-3s, play a role in hormone production. They contribute to cell health and can reduce inflammation, which is beneficial for hormonal balance.

Dietary Sources: Fatty fish (salmon, mackerel), chia seeds, nuts.

The Role of Fiber: Hormonal Cleansing

Dietary fibers can help regulate estrogen levels by facilitating their elimination through the digestive system. Sufficient fiber intake is associated with better hormonal balance.

Dietary Sources: Vegetables, fruits, whole grains, legumes.

Vitamins and Minerals: Microscopic Support

Vitamins like B6, vitamin E, and minerals like magnesium play a role in hormonal regulation.

Dietary Sources: Avocados (vitamin E), bananas (vitamin B6), spinach (magnesium).

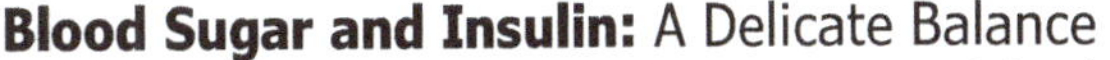

Blood Sugar and Insulin: A Delicate Balance
Maintaining stable blood sugar is crucial for hormonal balance. Low glycemic index foods and fiber-rich diets can help regulate insulin. Dietary Sources: Non-starchy vegetables, whole grains, legumes.

Omega-3s and Hormonal Health

Omega-3 fatty acids are recognized for their beneficial effects on hormonal health and inflammation. For those who wish to deepen their knowledge on the subject, here are some key references:

• Chang, Chuchun L., and Deckelbaum, Richard J. (2013). "Omega-3 Fatty Acids: Structures, Synthesis, and Nutrition." Current Opinion in Lipidology. This study explores the mechanisms by which omega-3s can contribute to the prevention of cardiovascular diseases.
• Marton, L. T., et al. (2019). "Omega-3 Fatty Acids and Inflammatory Processes: from Molecules to Man." International Journal of Molecular Sciences. This article reviews the anti-inflammatory effects of omega-3s, particularly in the context of inflammatory bowel diseases.
• Holm, T., et al. (2001). "Omega-3 Fatty Acid Treatment in Heart Transplant Recipients." Transplantation. This research examines the impact of omega-3s on inflammatory balance in patients who have undergone heart transplantation.
• Roman, A., et al. (2006). "Omega-3 Fatty Acids and Pregnancy." American Journal of Obstetrics and Gynecology. This study looks at the effects of omega-3s on the production of prostaglandins in decidual cells during pregnancy.
• Madison, A. A., et al. (2021). "Omega-3 Fatty Acids and Stress-Induced Immune Dysregulation: Implications for Wound Healing." Molecular Psychiatry. This article discusses the influence of omega-3s on stress, inflammation, and mental health.
• Hosny, M., et al. (2013). "Omega-3 Fatty Acids in Critical Care Medicine: New Approaches." The Egyptian Journal of Critical Care Medicine. This publication evaluates the safety and effectiveness of omega-3s in critical care medicine.
• Kim, J., et al. (2014). "Combination of Omega-3 Fatty Acids and Ursodeoxycholic Acid in the Treatment of Nonalcoholic Steatohepatitis." Experimental & Molecular Medicine. This study explores the combined effect of omega-3s and ursodeoxycholic acid on nonalcoholic steatohepatitis.

[...]

These references can be consulted for those who wish to understand in depth the mechanisms by which omega-3s influence our health. For our program, we will integrate omega-3s through foods such as fatty fish, flaxseed, nuts, and quality vegetable oils, to benefit from their positive effects on hormonal balance and inflammation reduction.

Nutritional Programs by Age Group

30-39 years: Focus on Fertility and Early Prevention

At this stage of life, a nutrient-rich diet is essential to support fertility and lay the foundations for long-term health. Foods rich in folic acid, iron, and omega-3 are particularly important.

Typical weekly menus:

Monday:
Breakfast: Protein green smoothie
Lunch: Mediterranean quinoa salad
Dinner: Baked salmon and seasonal vegetables

Tuesday:
Breakfast: Red berry porridge with chia seeds
Lunch: Chicken and roasted vegetable bowl
Dinner: Lentil curry and brown rice

Wednesday:
Breakfast: Avocado toast and poached egg
Lunch: Vegetarian wrap and green salad
Dinner: Grilled trout and sweet potato puree

Thursday:
Breakfast: Greek yogurt, homemade granola, and honey Lunch: Niçoise salad
Dinner: Herb-marinated chicken and quinoa

Friday:
Breakfast: Banana pancakes and maple syrup
Lunch: Tuna sandwich and raw vegetables
Dinner: Vegetable lasagna

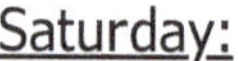

Saturday:
Breakfast: Spinach and feta omelette
Lunch: Falafel Buddha bowl
Dinner: White fish en papillote and herb rice

Sunday:
Breakfast: Whole English muffins and jam
Lunch: Pesto pasta salad with chicken
Dinner: Vegetable soup and whole bread

Each meal is designed to be balanced, nutrient-rich, and tailored to fertility and early prevention needs. You can repeat this pattern by changing the ingredients and recipes to create variety throughout the month.

40-49 Years: Managing Metabolism and Hormonal Changes
The forties can bring metabolic and hormonal changes, making weight management and hormonal balance more challenging. A diet rich in fiber, lean proteins, and cruciferous vegetables can help.

Typical Weekly Menus:

Monday:
Breakfast: Vegetable omelet with spinach, tomatoes, and mushrooms.
Lunch: Lentil salad with avocado, cherry tomatoes, and balsamic vinaigrette.
Dinner: Grilled chicken fillet, steamed broccoli, and baked sweet potato.

Tuesday:
Breakfast: Berry protein smoothie with chia seeds.
Lunch: Whole rice bowl with black beans, corn, salsa, and guacamole.
Dinner: White fish en papillote with fennel and carrots, accompanied by quinoa.

Wednesday:
Breakfast: Greek yogurt with sugar-free granola and fresh fruits.
Lunch: Turkey wrap with lettuce, tomato, cucumber, and hummus.
Dinner: Vegetarian chili with a variety of beans and vegetables, served with brown rice.

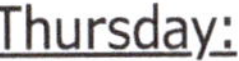

Thursday:
Breakfast: Oat porridge with apple, cinnamon, and nuts.
Lunch: Greek salad with grilled chicken.
Dinner: Tofu and Asian vegetable stir-fry with buckwheat noodles.

Friday:
Breakfast: Almond flour pancakes with pure maple syrup.
Lunch: Quinoa salad with spinach, nuts, goat cheese, and olive oil dressing.
Dinner: Vegetable curry with coconut milk and basmati rice.

Saturday:
Breakfast: Avocado toasts and scrambled eggs.
Lunch: Lentil soup and grilled cheese sandwich on whole bread.
Dinner: Grilled lamb chops with asparagus and celery root purée.

Sunday:
Breakfast: Green smoothie with spinach, cucumber, apple, lemon, and ginger.
Lunch: Mediterranean bowl with falafels, tabbouleh, hummus, and tzatziki.
Dinner: Vegetable lasagna with a green salad.

50-60 Years: Anti-Aging Nutrition and Maintaining Bone Density This period of life is crucial for the prevention of osteoporosis and maintaining cellular health. Foods rich in calcium, vitamin D, and antioxidants are a priority.

Typical Weekly Menus:

Monday:
Breakfast: Berry bowl with cottage cheese and a drizzle of honey.
Lunch: Kale salad with grilled chicken, avocado, and sunflower seeds.
Dinner: Baked salmon with sautéed spinach and quinoa.

Tuesday:
Breakfast: Red fruit smoothie with calcium-enriched almond milk.
Lunch: Open tuna sandwich with arugula salad and tomatoes on whole bread.
Dinner: Ratatouille with grilled tofu and brown rice.

Wednesday:
Breakfast: Muesli with nuts and dried fruits with almond milk.
Lunch: Niçoise salad with tuna, hard-boiled eggs, green beans, and olives.
Dinner: Roasted chicken with root vegetables and a small lamb's lettuce salad.

Thursday:
Breakfast: Rye toasts with fresh cheese and cucumber slices.
Lunch: Bulgur bowl with grilled vegetables and hummus.
Dinner: Coral lentil soup with spinach and whole bread.

Friday:
Breakfast: Poached eggs with spinach on grilled whole bread.
Lunch: Quinoa salad with beets, nuts, and goat cheese.
Dinner: Cod fillet en papillote with cherry tomatoes and olives, accompanied by bulgur.

Saturday:
Breakfast: Berry smoothie bowl with banana and chia seeds.
Lunch: Avocado tartine with soft-boiled egg and pumpkin seeds on whole bread.
Dinner: Stuffed eggplants with quinoa and vegetables, with homemade tomato sauce.

Sunday:
Breakfast: Buckwheat pancakes with unsweetened apple compote.
Lunch: White bean salad with tuna, red onion, and parsley.
Dinner: Winter vegetable stew with turkey pieces and pearl barley.

These menus are designed to be balanced and adapted to the specific nutritional needs of each age group, focusing on key nutrients for each life stage.

Weight Management

Introduction

Weight management is a personal and unique challenge for every woman. This chapter explores strategies for weight loss, gain, and maintenance, tailored to the specific needs of each age group. We emphasize the importance of caloric balance and share inspiring testimonials, accompanied by practical illustrations.

Weight Loss Strategies

Caloric Balance: The key to weight loss is to consume fewer calories than our body burns. This can be achieved by reducing portions, choosing less caloric foods, and increasing physical activity.

Balanced Diet: A diet rich in vegetables, fruits, lean proteins, and whole grains can help reduce caloric intake while staying satiated and providing necessary nutrients.

Physical Activity: Regular exercise, whether cardio or strength training, increases caloric expenditure and is essential for sustainable weight loss.

Weight Gain Strategies

Controlled Caloric Increase: For those looking to gain weight, it's important to increase caloric intake healthily, favoring foods rich in calories but also in nutrients.

Nutrient-Dense Foods: Nuts, seeds, avocados, and whole dairy products are excellent options to increase caloric intake without resorting to junk food.

EResistance Exercises: Strength training helps build muscle mass, which is preferable to fat accumulation during weight gain.

Weight Maintenance Strategies

Monitoring Caloric Intake: Finding a balance between calories consumed and expended is crucial to maintain weight.

Intuitive Eating: Learning to listen to your body and recognize hunger and satiety signals can help regulate food intake without counting calories.
Exercise Routine: A regular exercise routine helps stabilize weight and improve overall health.

Importance of Caloric Balance

Understanding Metabolism: Metabolism naturally decreases with age, which can affect caloric needs. Understanding this process is essential to adjust caloric intake.

Tracking Tools: Apps and food diaries can be used to track caloric intake and physical activity, allowing better weight control.

Diversity of Experiences: Each story is unique, reflecting the diversity of life paths and female bodies.

Conclusion

Weight management is a personal journey that requires a personalized approach. By understanding caloric balance and adopting strategies tailored to their body and lifestyle, women can achieve and maintain their ideal weight at every stage of their life.

Supplements

Here are some examples of popular apps and food journals that can help track caloric intake and physical activity:

<u>MyFitnessPal:</u> One of the most popular food and exercise tracking apps. It has a vast food database and allows barcode scanning for easy food logging.

<u>Lose It!:</u> This app focuses on weight loss by allowing users to set goals and track calories and nutrients.

<u>FatSecret:</u> Offers a complete food diary, physical activity tracking, and community support. It also includes a barcode scanner for foods.

<u>Cronometer:</u> An app that allows for more precise tracking of micronutrients, in addition to calories and physical activity.

<u>Yazio:</u> Offers a food diary, calorie tracking, and personalized advice to help achieve weight goals.

<u>SparkPeople:</u> In addition to food and exercise tracking, SparkPeople provides resources such as recipes and meal plans.

<u>Noom:</u> Uses a psychological approach to help change eating and lifestyle habits. It combines food tracking with daily lessons and coaching.

<u>Fitbit:</u> Known for its activity tracking devices, the Fitbit app also allows for food tracking and community connection for support.

<u>Fooducate:</u> Educates users on the quality of the foods they consume, in addition to tracking calories.

<u>Lifesum:</u> Offers meal plans and recipes, in addition to tracking food and exercise, to help achieve various health goals.

These apps can vary in terms of features, food databases, integration with other devices and apps, and tracking methods. It's important to choose an app that best matches the user's needs and preferences.

Weight Loss Journal

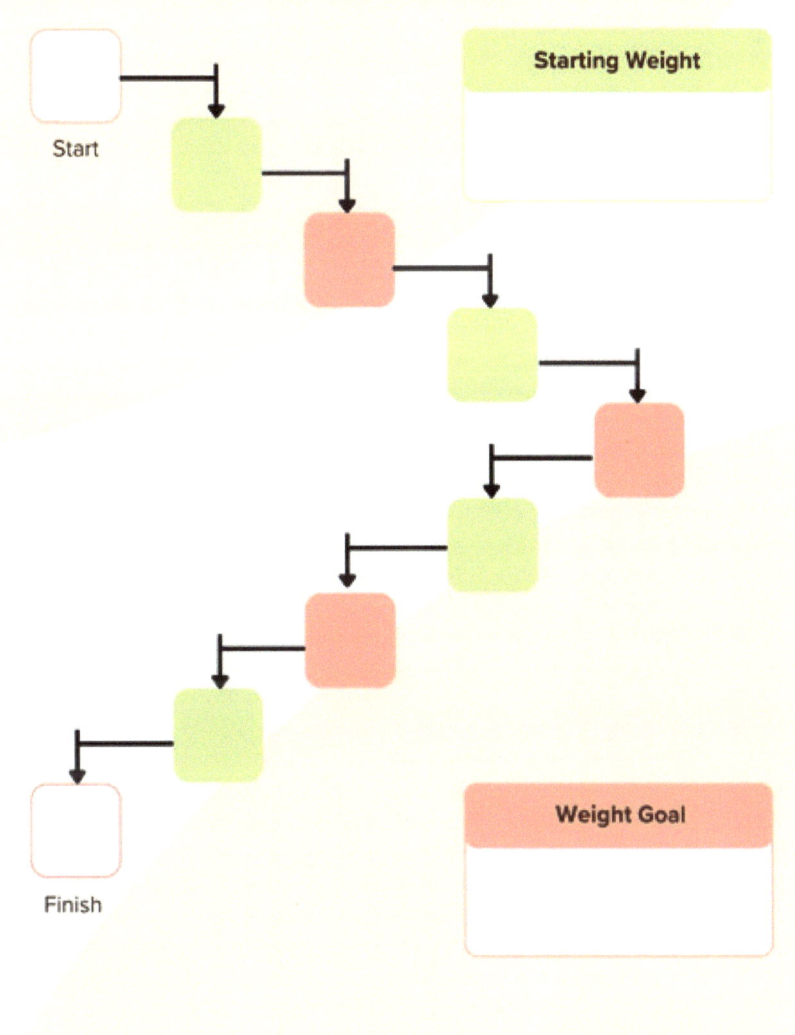

Mental Well-being and Nutrition

Introduction

The connection between nutrition and mental health is undeniable. This chapter explores how a balanced diet can support emotional well-being, and how practices such as relaxation and yoga can contribute to better mental health.

Foods that Support Emotional Well-being

Brain Nutrition:
Foods rich in omega-3 fatty acids, like salmon and chia seeds, support brain function and can improve mood.

Antioxidants and Mood:
Colorful fruits and vegetables, rich in antioxidants, protect brain cells from oxidative damage and can help reduce symptoms of depression.

Probiotics and Mental Health:
Fermented foods like yogurt, kefir, and sauerkraut contain probiotics that can have a positive impact on mental health by improving gut health.

B-Complex Vitamins:
B vitamins, particularly folate and B12 found in leafy green vegetables and lean meats, are essential for the production of mood-related neurotransmitters.

Relaxation and Yoga Exercises Conscious Breathing:
Breathing techniques like Pranayama can reduce stress and promote relaxation.

Meditation:
Mindfulness meditation can help reduce anxiety and improve mood by promoting presence and awareness.

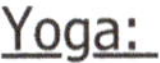

Yoga:
Regular yoga practice can decrease stress levels, improve flexibility and strength, and contribute to better emotional regulation.

Yoga Sequences for Mental Well-being

Gentle Yoga:
Gentle and restorative sequences, such as Yin Yoga or Hatha Yoga, are ideal for starting or ending the day with serenity.

Dynamic Yoga:
 More dynamic styles, like Vinyasa or Ashtanga, can be beneficial to elevate energy and improve concentration.

Specific Postures:
Postures like the lotus position (Padmasana) or child's pose (Balasana) are known for their calming effect on the mind.

"Mood-boosting" Foods

Dark Chocolate:
Rich in flavonoids, dark chocolate can improve brain circulation and mood.

Green Tea: Containing L-theanine, green tea can help promote relaxation without drowsiness.

Whole Grains: Complex carbohydrates from whole grains promote the production of serotonin, often called the happiness hormone.

Conclusion

A balanced diet, rich in essential nutrients, and a regular practice of relaxation and yoga can play a crucial role in maintaining mental health. By integrating these elements into daily routines, women can enhance their emotional well-being and quality of life.

Superfoods for Women

Introduction

Superfoods are nutrient-rich foods that offer significant health benefits. For women, certain superfoods can provide specific benefits, such as improving hormonal health, preventing diseases, and boosting energy and vitality.

Superfoods and Their Benefits

Goji Berries: Rich in vitamins, minerals, and antioxidants, Goji berries are renowned for their ability to boost energy and mental performance.

Chia Seeds: An excellent source of omega-3, fiber, and protein, chia seeds can help regulate blood sugar and maintain a healthy weight.

Spinach: Spinach is loaded with iron, essential for preventing anemia, especially in women of childbearing age.

Turmeric: Known for its anti-inflammatory properties, turmeric can help manage inflammation and menstrual pain.

Wild Salmon: A source of high-quality omega-3, wild salmon supports heart health and can help reduce the risk of chronic diseases.

Quinoa: Quinoa is a complete source of plant-based protein and is rich in fiber, iron, and magnesium.

Matcha Tea: Matcha is a powerful antioxidant that can help protect against heart disease and certain cancers.

Sweet Potato: Rich in vitamin A and fiber, sweet potatoes promote healthy skin and can help regulate blood sugar.

Walnuts: These nuts are a good source of omega-3 fatty acids and antioxidants, beneficial for brain health and preventing heart diseases.

Oats: Oats are rich in soluble fiber, which can help lower cholesterol and promote digestive health.

How to Incorporate Superfoods into Your Diet

Smoothies: Add Goji berries, chia seeds, and matcha to smoothies for a nutritional boost.

Salads: Incorporate spinach, quinoa, and walnuts into salads for a nutrient-rich meal.

Main Dishes: Use wild salmon and sweet potatoes as main ingredients in meals for their health benefits.

Snacks: Oats can be transformed into energy bars or granola for healthy and convenient snacks.

Conclusion

Superfoods can play a key role in enhancing the health and well-being of women. By regularly incorporating them into their diet, women can benefit from their nutritious and protective properties. This chapter encourages women to discover and experiment with these powerful foods to enhance their overall health.

Recipes with Superfoods

These recipes are simple, nutritious, and delicious, and they can be easily adapted based on personal preferences or dietary restrictions. They are designed to incorporate superfoods into your daily regimen, thus improving overall health and well-being.

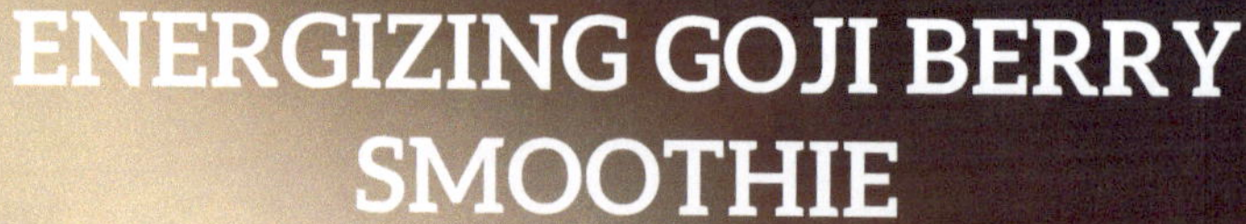

ENERGIZING GOJI BERRY SMOOTHIE

- **1 tablespoon of dried goji berries**
- **1 ripe banana**
- **1/2 cup of strawberries**
- **1 cup of almond milk or coconut milk**
- **1 teaspoon of honey or maple syrup (optional)**
- **Ice cubes**

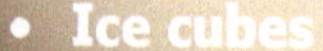

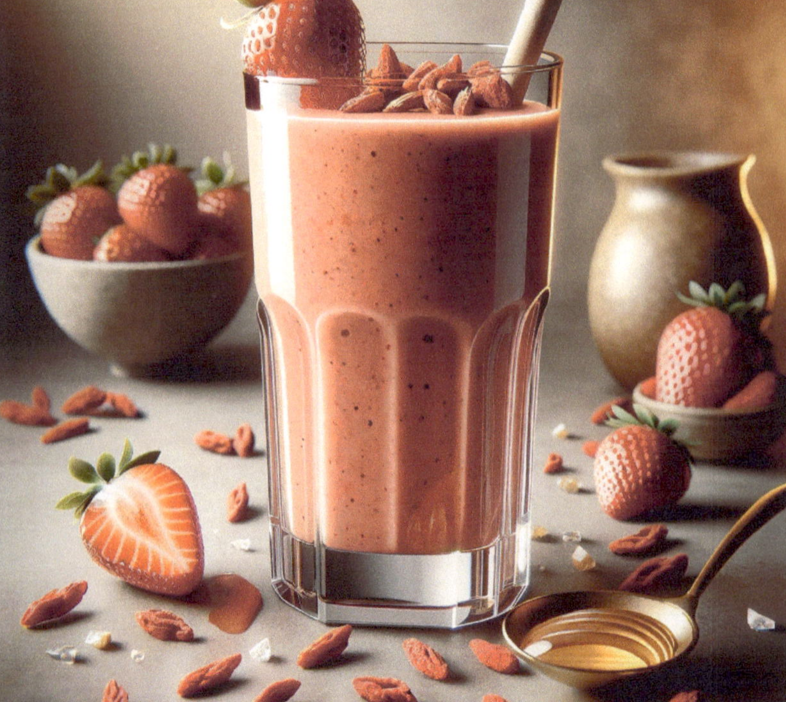

Instructions:

- **- Soak the goji berries in hot water for 10 minutes to rehydrate them.**
- **In a blender, combine the drained goji berries, the banana, strawberries, almond milk, and honey.**
- **Add ice cubes and blend until smooth.**

Serve immediately for a natural energy boost.

CHIA SEED PUDDING

3 tablespoons of chia seeds
1 cup of almond milk or coconut milk
1 teaspoon of vanilla extract
1 tablespoon of maple syrup or honey
Fresh fruit for garnish

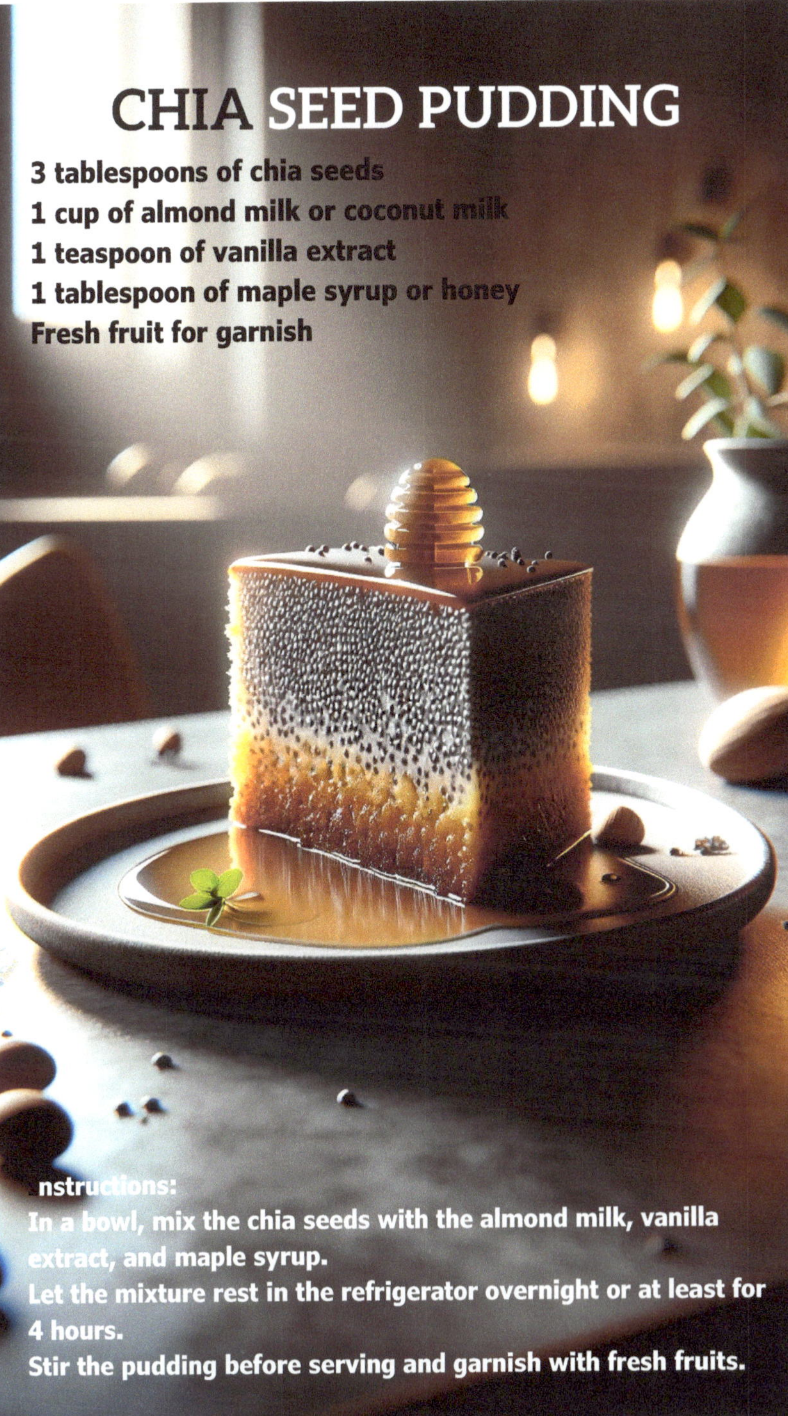

Instructions:
In a bowl, mix the chia seeds with the almond milk, vanilla extract, and maple syrup.
Let the mixture rest in the refrigerator overnight or at least for 4 hours.
Stir the pudding before serving and garnish with fresh fruits.

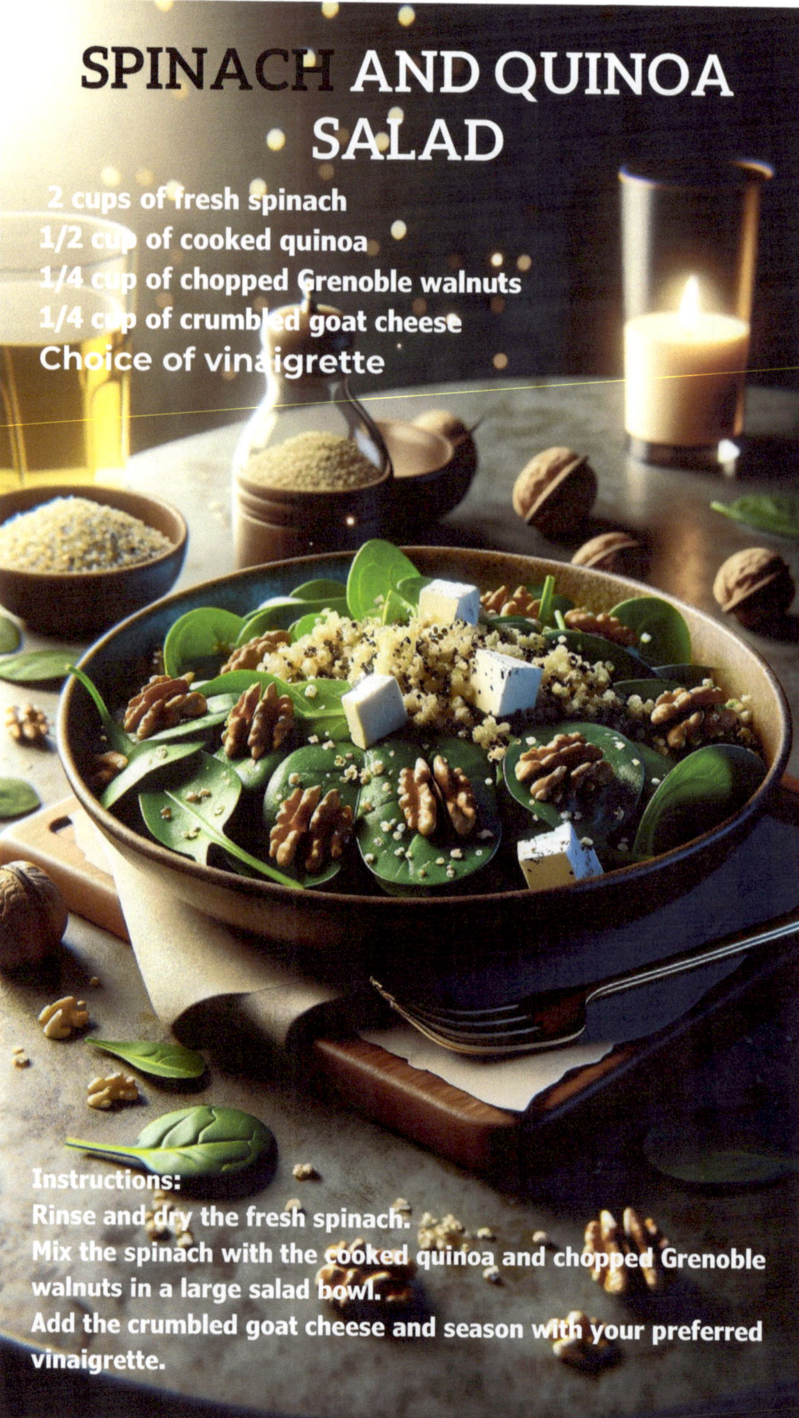

SPINACH AND QUINOA SALAD

2 cups of fresh spinach
1/2 cup of cooked quinoa
1/4 cup of chopped Grenoble walnuts
1/4 cup of crumbled goat cheese
Choice of vinaigrette

Instructions:
Rinse and dry the fresh spinach.
Mix the spinach with the cooked quinoa and chopped Grenoble walnuts in a large salad bowl.
Add the crumbled goat cheese and season with your preferred vinaigrette.

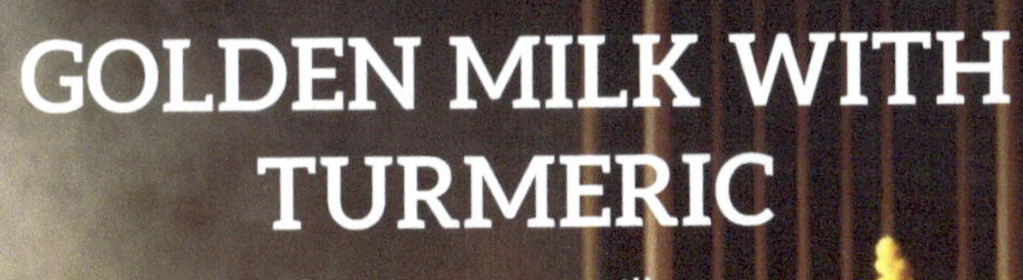

GOLDEN MILK WITH TURMERIC

1 cup of almond milk or coconut milk
1 teaspoon of turmeric powder
1/2 teaspoon of cinnamon powder
1 pinch of ground black pepper (for absorption)
1 teaspoon of honey or maple syrup

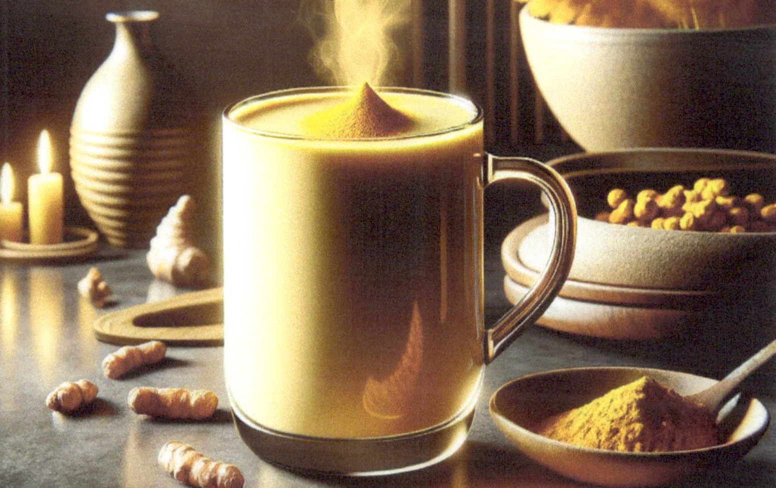

Instructions:
In a saucepan, heat the milk with the turmeric, cinnamon, and black pepper.
Bring to a boil, then reduce the heat and let simmer for a few minutes.
Remove from the heat, add honey or maple syrup, and mix well.
Serve hot for a comforting and anti-inflammatory drink.

Nutrition sportive pour les femmes activesSports Nutrition for Active Women

Introduction

Nutrition plays a crucial role in athletic performance and recovery. This chapter focuses on the specific needs of active women, emphasizing pre- and post-workout nutrition, hydration, and recovery.

Pre-Workout Nutrition

Goal:To provide energy and prevent muscle fatigue.

Recommended Snacks: Banana with almond butter, Greek yogurt with berries, avocado toast.

Timing: Consume 30 to 60 minutes before exercising. Key

Nutrients: Carbohydrates for energy, proteins for the prevention of muscle breakdown.

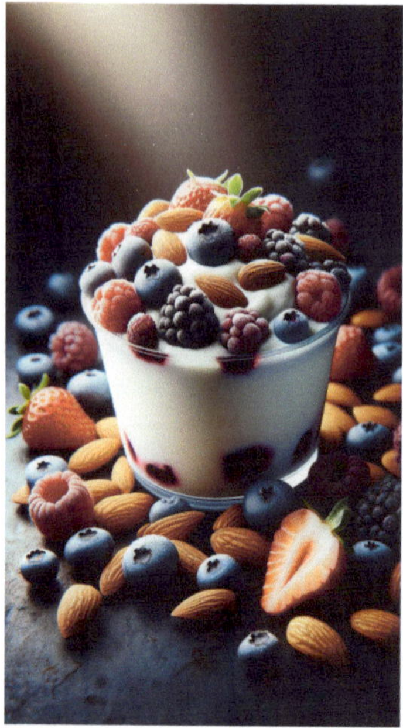

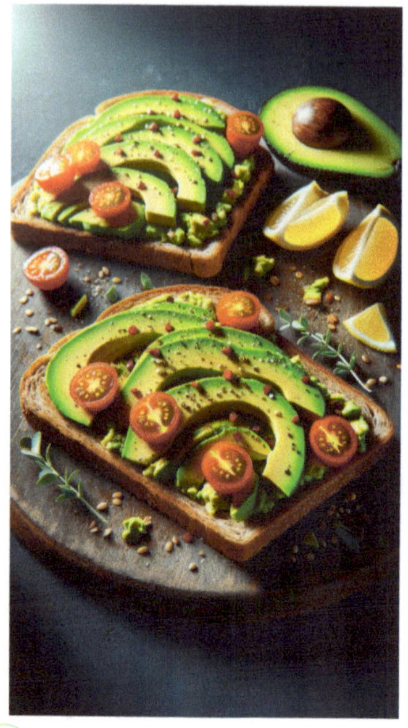

Post-Workout Nutrition

<u>Goal:</u> To aid muscle recovery and replenish energy stores.

<u>Recommended Snacks:</u> Protein smoothie with spinach, fruits, and chia seeds; vegetable omelet; quinoa with grilled chicken.

<u>Timing:</u> Within 45 minutes following exercise.

<u>Key Nutrients:</u> Proteins for muscle repair, carbohydrates to replenish glycogen.

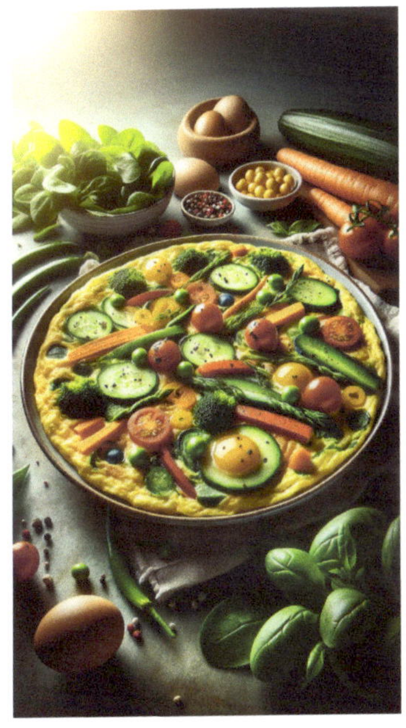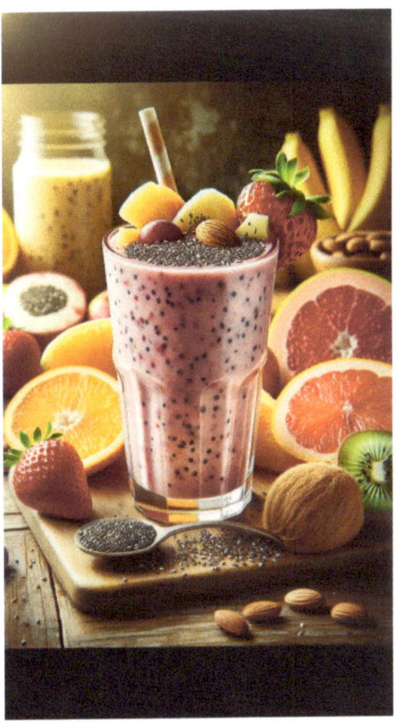

Hydration and Recovery

<u>Hydration :</u> Drinking water before, during, and after exercise is crucial. Hydration with electrolyte drinks can be beneficial after intense or prolonged sessions.

<u>Recovery:</u> Amino acids, such as L-glutamine found in protein-rich foods, can aid in muscle recovery. Anti-inflammatory foods like salmon and berries can also reduce muscle soreness.

Conclusion

Proper nutrition is vital for active women to maximize their performance and recovery. By understanding and applying these sports nutrition principles, women can improve their endurance, strength, and overall recovery.

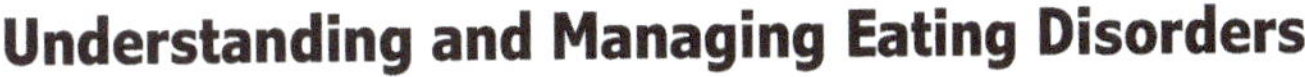

Understanding and Managing Eating Disorders

Introduction

Eating disorders are serious conditions that affect both physical and mental health. This chapter aims to raise awareness about the early detection of eating disorders and the importance of professional help.

Signs of Detection

Common Symptoms:
Excessive preoccupation with weight and body shape.
Severe dietary restriction or episodes of overeating.
Compensatory behaviors such as fasting, misuse of laxatives, or excessive exercise.
Mood swings, social withdrawal, and low self-esteem.

Physical Signs:
Significant weight loss or gain.
Chronic digestive issues.
Fatigue and muscle weakness.
In women, menstrual irregularities or the absence of periods.

Importance of Professional Help

Accès aux Soins:Access to Care:
Encourage individuals suffering from eating disorders to seek professional help at the first signs.
Management may include behavioral therapies, nutritional support, and if necessary, medical treatment.

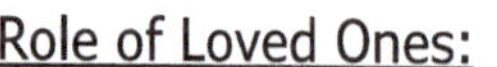

<u>Role of Loved Ones:</u>
Loved ones play a crucial role in providing support and encouragement to seek help. Being attentive, avoiding judgment, and encouraging the individual to talk about their struggles.

Conclusion

Early recognition of eating disorders and prompt intervention are essential for a successful recovery. This chapter aims to educate and provide useful resources for those affected by these conditions, as well as for their loved ones.

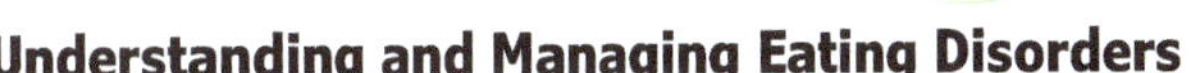

Understanding and Managing Eating Disorders

Introduction

A well-structured exercise program is crucial for maintaining good physical and mental health. This chapter offers simple exercises suited for different age groups, with a 28-day program to encourage a regular physical activity routine.

Simple Exercises for Each Age Group

30-39 years:
Focus: Muscle strengthening and cardio. Exercise Examples: Squats, modified push-ups, light jogging, or brisk walking.

40-49 years:
Focus: Balance and flexibility. Exercise Examples: Yoga, Pilates, cycling.

50-60 years:
Focus: Low impact and maintaining bone density. Exercise Examples: Nordic walking, swimming, gentle resistance exercises.

28-Day Program

Week 1: Introduction to basic exercises, focusing on familiarization.

Monday: Brisk Walking
Duration: 20 minutes. Focus: Warming up the body, improving cardiovascular endurance.
Tuesday: Basic Squats
Repetitions: 2 sets of 10. Focus: Strengthening legs and glutes.
Wednesday: Rest or Light Walking
Thursday: Modified Push-Ups (on knees)
Repetitions: 2 sets of 8. Focus: Upper body strengthening.
Friday: General Stretching
Duration: 15 minutes. Focus: Flexibility and recovery.
Saturday and Sunday: Leisure Activity
Example: Bike ride, gentle swimming.

Week 2: Gradual increase in intensity and duration.

Monday: Brisk Walking
Duration: 30 minutes.
Tuesday: Alternating Squats and Lunges
Repetitions: 2 sets of 12 for each exercise.
Wednesday: Active Rest
Example: Gentle yoga.
Thursday: Modified Push-Ups and Planks
Push-ups: 2 sets of 10. Planks: 2 times 30 seconds.
Friday: Stretching and Mobility
Duration: 20 minutes.
Weekend: Hiking or Swimming Duration: 45 minutes to 1 hour

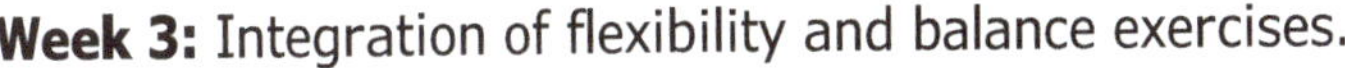

Week 3: Integration of flexibility and balance exercises.

Monday: Basic Pilates
Duration: 30 minutes.
Tuesday: Light Strength Circuit Include exercises like squats, push-ups, and resistance band exercises.
Wednesday: Balance Yoga
Duration: 30 minutes.
Thursday: Moderate Cardio
Example: Cycling, dancing.
Friday: Stretching and Relaxation Duration: 20 minutes.
Weekend: Outdoor Activity Example: Hiking, kayaking

Week 4: Consolidation of skills and introduction of variations to maintain engagement.

Monday: Brisk Walking Intervals Alternating between brisk walking and normal walking.
Tuesday: Combined Circuit Combination of squats, lunges, and arm exercises with light weights.
Wednesday: Dynamic Yoga A more intense session to improve strength and flexibility.
Thursday: Boxing or Cardio Dance A fun session to boost endurance.
Friday: Advanced Pilates
Focus on core strength and balance.
Weekend: Free Choice Encourage choosing an enjoyable physical activity

Menus and Meal Plans for 28 Days

Introduction

This chapter provides balanced daily menus for three meals a day, with examples of dishes and their caloric intake, including drinks. The recipes are designed to be simple, nutritious, and suitable for an active lifestyle.

Daily Menu Examples:

Day 1

Breakfast: Spinach and Feta Omelette (200 calories) Berry and Greek Yogurt Smoothie (150 calories) Green Tea (0 calories)

Lunch: Grilled Vegetable Quinoa Salad (350 calories) Lemon and Mint Infused Water (0 calories)

Dinner: Grilled Salmon Fillet with Asparagus (400 calories) Brown Rice (200 calories) Red Wine (125 calories)

Day 2

Breakfast: Fresh Fruit Porridge with Nuts (250 calories) Black Coffee (5 calories)

Lunch: Chicken and Avocado Wrap (400 calories) Sparkling Water with a Slice of Lemon (0 calories)

Dinner: Vegetable and Tofu Curry (350 calories) Basmati Rice (180 calories) Unsweetened Iced Tea (0 calories)

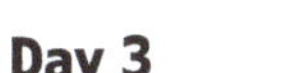

Day 3

<u>Breakfast:</u> Green Smoothie (Spinach, Apple, Cucumber) (180 calories) Whole Grain Toast with Almond Butter (150 calories)

<u>Lunch:</u> Niçoise Salad (300 calories) Still Water (0 calories)

<u>Dinner:</u> Zucchini Spaghetti with Shrimp (350 calories) Green Salad (50 calories) Glass of White Wine (120 calories)

Day 4

<u>PBreakfast:</u> Banana and Oatmeal Pancakes (250 calories) Fresh Orange Juice (110 calories)

<u>Lunch:</u> Lentil Soup (220 calories) Whole Grain Bread (80 calories) Cucumber Infused Water (0 calories)

<u>Dinner:</u> Herb-Roasted Chicken with Root Vegetables (450 calories) Green Salad with Light Dressing (70 calories) Sparkling Water (0 calories)

Day 5

<u>PBreakfast:</u> Greek Yogurt with Honey and Granola (300 calories) Milk Coffee (50 calories)

<u>Lunch:</u> Tuna Sandwich and Salad (350 calories) Unsweetened Iced Tea (0 calories)

<u>Dinner:</u> Vegetable Lasagna (400 calories) Light Caesar Salad (150 calories) Glass of Red Wine (125 calories)

Day 6

<u>Breakfast:</u> Red Fruit Protein Smoothie (200 calories) Whole Grain Toast with Avocado (200 calories)

<u>Lunch:</u> Vegetable, Quinoa, and Tofu Buddha Bowl (400 calories) Raspberry Infused Water (0 calories)

<u>Dinner:</u> White Fish en Papillote with Seasonal Vegetables (350 calories) Quinoa (150 calories) Sparkling Water with Lemon (0 calories)

Day 7

<u>PBreakfast:</u> Scrambled Eggs on Whole Grain Toast (250 calories) Fresh Apple Juice (120 calories)

<u>Lunch:</u> Grilled Chicken and Avocado Salad (350 calories) Still Water (0 calories)

<u>Dinner:</u> Mushroom Risotto (400 calories) Arugula Salad (50 calories) Glass of White Wine (120 calories)

<u>Day 8</u>

<u>Breakfast:</u> Fresh Fruit Bowl with Yogurt and Chia Seeds (300 calories) Green Tea (0 calories)

<u>Lunch:</u> Chickpea and Grilled Vegetable Salad (350 calories) Lime Infused Water (0 calories)

<u>Dinner:</u> Grilled Tuna Steak with Quinoa Salad (450 calories) Steamed Vegetables (50 calories) Sparkling Water (0 calories)

Day 9

<u>Breakfast:</u> Whole Grain English Muffins with Peanut Butter (250 calories) Black Coffee (5 calories)

<u>Lunch:</u> Pumpkin and Carrot Soup (200 calories) Grilled Whole Grain Bread (80 calories) Still Water (0 calories)

<u>Dinner:</u> Chicken Curry with Vegetables (400 calories) Basmati Rice (200 calories) Unsweetened Iced Tea (0 calories)

Day 10

<u>Breakfast:</u> Spinach, Banana, and Protein Smoothie (250 calories) Rice Cakes with Avocado (150 calories)

<u>Lunch:</u> Greek Salad with Feta and Olives (300 calories) Lemon Flavored Water (0 calories)

<u>Dinner:</u> Vegetarian Lasagna (400 calories) Green Salad (50 calories) Glass of Red Wine (125 calories)

Day11

<u>Breakfast:</u> Poached Eggs on Whole Grain Toast (300 calories) Tomato Juice (50 calories)

<u>Lunch:</u> Vegetarian Wrap with Hummus and Raw Veggies (350 calories) Sparkling Water with a Slice of Lemon (0 calories)

<u>Dinner:</u> Salmon en Papillote with Seasonal Vegetables (400 calories) Couscous (200 calories) Herbal Tea (0 calories)

Day 12

Breakfast: Blueberry and almond porridge (250 calories)
Black tea (0 calories)

Lunch: Lentil and roasted vegetable salad (350 calories)
Mint-infused water (0 calories)

Dinner: Grilled chicken and vegetable skewers (400 calories)
Brown rice (200 calories) Sparkling water (0 calories)

Day 13

Breakfast: Green smoothie (kale, apple, cucumber) (180 calories) Whole grain bread with fresh cheese (200 calories)

Lunch: Buddha bowl with quinoa, avocado, and tofu (400 calories) Raspberry-infused water (0 calories)

Dinner: Seafood spaghetti (350 calories) Arugula salad (50 calories) Glass of white wine (120 calories)

Day14

Breakfast: Whole wheat waffles with maple syrup (300 calories) coffee with milk (50 calories)

Lunch: Chicken and raw vegetable sandwich (350 calories) Unsweetened iced tea (0 calories)

Dinner: Vegetarian chili (400 calories) Whole rice (200 calories) Orange-flavored water (0 calories)

These menus are designed to offer a balance between flavors, nutrition, and ease of preparation, considering daily caloric and nutritional needs. They can be adapted according to personal preferences and the seasons.

For the following days, continue to vary the menus by alternating between the proposed options for breakfast, lunch, and dinner. Ensure to include a variety of proteins, vegetables, fruits, and whole grains. Beverages should remain primarily unsweetened and low in calories.

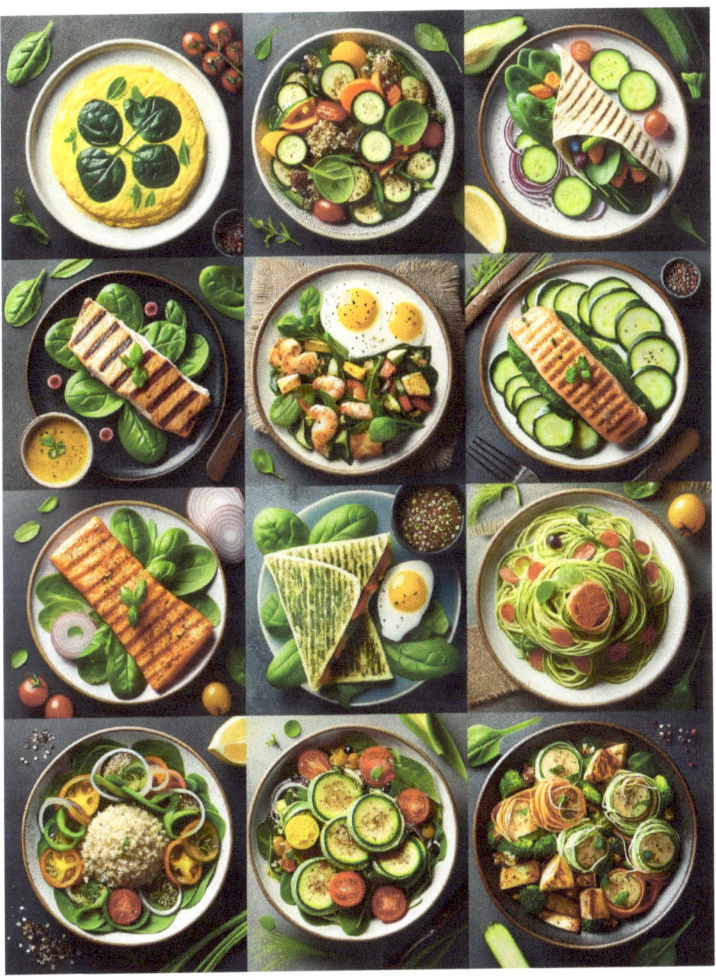

DAY	BREAKFAST	LUNCH	DINNER
1	Spinach Omelette 200 Cal.	Quinoa Salad 350 Cal.	Grilled Salmon Asparagus 400 Cal.
2	Fruit Porridge 250 Cal.	Chicken Wrap 400 Cal.	Végetables curry 180 Cal.
3	Green Smoothie 200 Cal.	Niçoise salad 300 Cal.	Zucchini Spaghetti 350 Cal.
4	Banana Pancake 250 Cal.	Lentil soup 220 Cal.	Herb Roasted Chicken 450 Cal.
5	Greek Yogurt with Honey 300 Cal.	Tuna Sandwich 350 Cal.	Vegetable Lasagna 400 Cal.
6	Red Fruit Smoothie 200 Cal.	Buddha Bowl Vegetables 400 Cal.	White Fish in Papillote 350 Cal.
7	Scrambled Eggs 250 Cal.	Grilled Chicken Salad 350 Cal.	Mushroom Risotto 400 Cal.

DAY	BREAKFAST	LUNCH	DINNER
8	Berry fruit yogurt **300 Cal.**	Chickpea Salad **350 Cal.**	Grilled Tuna Steak **450 Cal.**
9	Fruit Porridge (**250 Cal.**	Chicken Wrap **400 Cal.**	Vegetables curry **180 Cal.**
10	Green Smoothie **250 Cal.**	Greek Salad **300 Cal.**	Vegetarian Lasagna **400 Cal.**
11	Poached Eggs **300 Cal.**	Vegetarian Wrap **350 Cal.**	Salmon en Papillote **400 Cal.**
12	Blueberry Porridge **250 Cal.**	Lentil Salad **350 Cal.**	Chicken Skewers **400 Cal.**
13	Green Smoothie **180 Cal.**	Quinoa Buddha Bowl **400 Cal.**	Seafood Spaghetti **350 Cal.**
14	Waffles with Maple Syrup **300 Cal.**	Chicken Sandwich **350 Cal.**	Vegetarian Chili **400 Cal.**

DAY	BREAKFAST	LUNCH	DINNER
15	...... Cal.	...... Cal.	...... Cal.
16	...... Cal.	...... Cal.	...... Cal.
17	...... Cal.	...... Cal.	...... Cal.
18	...... Cal.	...... Cal.	...... Cal.
19	...... Cal.	...... Cal.	...... Cal.
20	...... Cal.	...... Cal.	.......Cal.
21	...... Cal.	...... Cal.	...... Cal.

DAY	BREAKFAST	LUNCH	DINNER
22	...... Cal.	...... Cal.	...... Cal.
23	...... Cal.	...... Cal.	...... Cal.
24	...... Cal.	...... Cal.	...... Cal.
25	...... Cal.	...... Cal.	...... Cal.
26	...... Cal.	...... Cal.	...... Cal.
27	...... Cal.	...... Cal.	.......Cal.
28	...... Cal.	...... Cal.	...... Cal.

Conclusion

Summary of Key Principles

This book has covered several essential aspects of nutrition and well-being, tailored to the specific needs of women at different stages of their lives. Here is a summary of the key principles:

Understanding the Basics of Nutrition: Knowledge of macronutrients, vitamins, minerals, and the importance of dietary balance is fundamental.

Hormonal Balance and Nutrition: Foods play a crucial role in hormonal regulation, especially through omega-3s, fiber, and antioxidants. Nutritional Programs by Age Group: Adapting diet according to age is essential to meet the body's changing needs.

Weight Management: Understanding caloric balance and strategies tailored for weight loss, gain, or maintenance is crucial.

Mental Well-being and Nutrition: A healthy diet significantly contributes to mental and emotional health.

Superfoods for Women: Certain foods offer specific health benefits for women's health.

Sports Nutrition: Diet influences athletic performance and recovery.

Understanding and Managing Eating Disorders: Early detection and intervention are key to effective management.

Physical Exercise Program: Regular physical activity complements good nutrition.

28-Day Menus and Meal Plans: Concrete examples to integrate these principles into daily life.

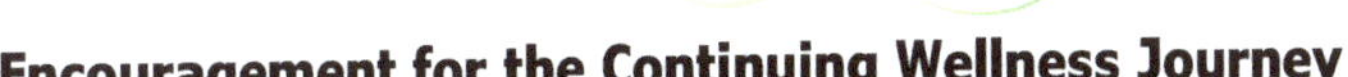

Encouragement for the Continuing Wellness Journey

Your journey towards optimal well-being does not stop at the last page of this book. Every day presents a new opportunity to make healthy choices and take care of yourself. Remember that small steps can lead to significant changes. Be patient with yourself and celebrate every success, no matter how small.

Success Stories

To inspire you, here are some testimonials from women who have transformed their lives through better nutrition and an active lifestyle:

Marie, 35 years old: "After following the advice in this book, I not only lost weight, but I also gained energy and self-confidence. It has incredibly changed my life."

Linda, 47 years old: "By adapting my diet to my hormonal needs, I managed to better handle my menopause symptoms. I feel more balanced and serene."

Sophie, 52 years old: "Thanks to the exercise programs and meal plans, I have strengthened my bones and improved my bone density. I feel stronger and younger."

These testimonials prove that no matter your age or circumstances, it is always possible to improve your health and well-being. We hope that this book will serve as a guide and inspiration on your path to a healthier and happier life.

Appendices

Glossary of Nutritional Terms

Macronutrients: Proteins, carbohydrates, and fats, which are the main components of our diet.

Micronutrients: Vitamins and minerals required in small amounts for various body functions.

Antioxidants: Compounds that protect cells against damage caused by free radicals.

Omega-3: Essential fatty acids beneficial for heart, brain, and hormonal health.

Fiber: Essential for good digestion and blood sugar regulation.

Probiotics: Beneficial bacteria that support gut health.

Blood Sugar: The level of sugar in the blood.

Metabolism: The set of chemical reactions in the body that transform or use energy.

Bone Density: A measure of the amount of minerals in the bones.

Calorie: A unit of measurement for the energy provided by food.

References and Scientific Sources

To ensure the reliability and accuracy of the information presented in this book, here is a list of the main scientific sources used:

Journal of Nutrition
American Journal of Clinical Nutrition
European Journal of Nutrition
International Journal of Behavioral Nutrition and Physical Activity
Nutrients
Harvard Health Publishing
Mayo Clinic Proceedings

Specific studies and research articles are cited throughout the book to support the claims made in each chapter.

Useful Contacts for Support and Guidance

For those seeking additional support or professional advice, here is a list of useful contacts:

Nutrition and Dietetics Associations: For personalized nutritional advice.
Eating Disorder Helplines: For immediate and confidential support.

Local Support Groups: To share experiences and advice with others who have similar goals.

Nutrition Research Institutes: For scientific information and up-to-date recommendations.

Fitness and Wellness Centers: For advice on physical exercise and overall well-being.

These resources can provide additional information, emotional support, and practical advice to help you on your wellness journey.